# REEDS
# FIRST AID
# HANDBOOK

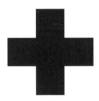

REEDS
Bloomsbury Publishing Plc
50 Bedford Square, London WC1B 3DP
29 Earlsfort Terrace, Dublin 2, Ireland

BLOOMSBURY and REEDS are trademarks of Bloomsbury Publishing Plc
First published in Great Britain 2024

A catalogue record for this book is available from the British Library
Library of Congress Cataloguing-in-Publication data has been applied for

ISBN: PB: 978-1-3994-0121-0;
ePub: 978-1-3994-0123-4;
ePDF: 978-1-3994-0122-7

2 4 6 8 10 9 7 5 3 1

Typeset in Myriad Light 9/11pt by carrdesignstudio.com

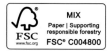

Printed and bound in UAE by Oriental Press

Note: While all reasonable care has been taken in preparation of this
publication, the authors and publisher accept no responsibility for
any errors or omissions or consequences ensuing upon the use of
the methods, information or products described in the book.

To find out more about our authors and books visit www.
bloomsbury.com and sign up for our newsletters.

# REEDS
# FIRST AID
# HANDBOOK

**Martin Thomas
& Olivia Davies**

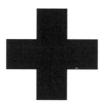

**R E E D S**

LONDON • OXFORD • NEW YORK • NEW DELHI • SYDNEY
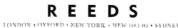

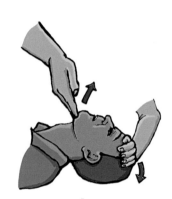

# CONTENTS

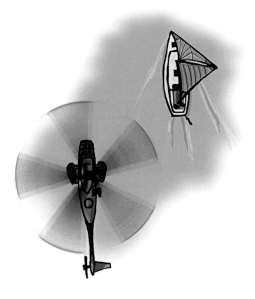

# Introduction

This book is written for anyone who sets sail on a vessel without a medic aboard – so most vessels at sea.

Although there is a limit on what can be done on a small boat, nevertheless with appropriate intervention as described in this handbook, the medical condition of a patient can be significantly improved and in some circumstances lives can even be saved.

Skippers and their crew, especially long distance sailors, are advised to attend a training course in first aid. Advice on more expert interventions (from giving someone fluids intravenously to inserting a chest drain) are not offered in this handbook. These manoeuvres are potentially hazardous if attempted by non-medics unfamiliar and untrained in such techniques.

For bigger boats with a larger crew and for those travelling long distances to remote areas, it is advisable to have aboard a crew member designated as responsible for medical care. This person might be a medic, a nurse or someone who has specifically trained in first aid and marine or wilderness medicine.

Martin Thomas
Olivia Davies

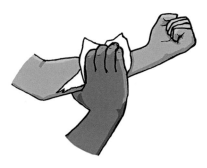

Before setting sail thought must be given to the medical care of the crew. The longer and more remote the voyage the more essential is detailed medical planning. The skipper must be aware of any health problems amongst those on board. If a crew member has a medical condition such as diabetes, epilepsy, hypertension, heart problems, allergies, asthma or other breathing problems then not only must they tell the skipper but they must also take adequate medication for the entire trip. If a crew member knows that they are likely to be seasick, they should take enough of their own preferred medication and not deplete the ship's stocks.

If the voyage is planned for parts of the world where immunisation is required, then seek medical advice beforehand. Leave plenty of time to get immunised – at least three months. Remember to arrange malarial prophylaxis and to start taking it in advance. A dental check-up is also sensible to avoid the misery of a dental abscess mid-ocean.

Any long distance sailor and certainly the skipper should attend a recognised course in first aid and basic medical procedures. A boat crossing any stretch of open sea should have two people aboard who can perform cardiopulmonary resuscitation (CPR). The boat must be furnished with a simple first aid manual and a larger more comprehensive medical manual.

Thought must be given as to which drugs and medical kit will be taken. The drugs and kit must be appropriate to the voyage planned and the crew aboard. Drugs are like nautical knots – the boat needs a few good ones that work well and are familiar to the crew.

Take details of a shore-based medical facility prepared to give long distance medical advice via telemedicine.

### Planning

Examples are MSOS (Medical Support Offshore) run by Dr Spike Briggs, PRAXES (Clipper Telemed) and Medaire. International MRCCs (Maritime Rescue Coordinate Centres) such as the one at Falmouth, UK, will also arrange medical advice. A satellite phone is the most convenient way of receiving such information or else use the Inmarsat-C messaging system. It is wise to take out medical insurance to include repatriation.

## *Prevention is better than cure*

A crew that is well fed and adequately rested will suffer fewer medical problems. This means regular proper meals and a well run watch system. Crew on a tidy vessel run 'shipshape and Bristol fashion', with a place for everything and everything in its place, will suffer fewer injuries.

Particular care must be taken when attending the anchor, the windlass or the engine. Crew should know and practice methods for reefing in heavy weather, for gybing, mast climbing and inspecting the propeller. Such familiarity will reduce the risk of a significant injury.

Crew should wear a lifejacket, a harness and clip on at night, in rough weather and when in the cockpit alone. It is wise to inform another crew member whenever going forward of the mast for any reason, especially at night. When cooking it is wise for crew to wear trousers, maybe an apron, and shoes. Crew below must beware, it is so easy to be thrown across the cabin. Remember: one hand for the boat and one for yourself.

In a reasonably small boat at sea, cold and fatigue can render crew members unable to function. The impact of this must not be underestimated. Fatigue can lead to poor decisions and errors that place the vessel in danger. Crew must wear clothing appropriate to the conditions. Good weatherproof outer garments are essential to keep out wind and water. Layering of clothing is the key to warmth. Wrap up in good time, even before the boat sets sail and certainly before the risk of getting wet. If a sailor is drenched then a change into dry clothes is essential. Wind chill on wet clothes can lead towards hypothermia.

Fatigue can creep up unnoticed, which is why certain occupations (lorry driver, airline pilot) have limited work hours. The key to avoiding fatigue is a good watch system for both the crew and the skipper. Anxious, inexperienced skippers can stay on deck too long and become tired and unreliable. Regular meals taken off watch, preferably hot, are good for morale and contribute to the effectiveness of the ship's company. Crew must take regular rest, food and drink (preferably not alcohol), so that when the crisis occurs they can deal with it judiciously.

## Seasickness

Every seafarer has been afflicted by seasickness at some time, but a crew member suffering from it can become unable to function thus reducing the number of effective crew to work the boat.

Motion sickness occurs when there is a disconnect between the body's perception of motion and the actual motion – the sensory conflict theory. Sickness can be caused by motion that is felt but not seen. This applies when down below where the eyes perceive no movement but the vestibular apparatus in the middle ear does. Early symptoms include lethargy, yawning, excess salivation and sweating. Then come fatigue, headache, dizziness and eventually nausea and vomiting.

## Prevention

Seasickness is another malady where prevention is important as there is no specific cure.

- ◆ Set out on the voyage rested, well hydrated and alcohol free.
- ◆ Avoid alcohol for 12 hours prior to sailing.
- ◆ By setting out in calmer weather and perhaps going to a quiet anchorage for the first night, a process of acclimatisation can begin. Finding one's 'sea legs' takes most people no more than 48 hours.
- ◆ Ginger has been shown to be helpful in warding off the malady. Ginger taken as capsules or sachets or as ginger biscuits may help. Other remedies recommended, such as cola drinks or warm tea, probably act solely through the placebo effect.

## Medication

Medication designed to prevent seasickness should be taken the evening before departure or earlier. Not to take medication until symptoms appear is a grave error. Attempting to treat sickness once it has occurred is the least effective option and rarely works. So much better to take the tablets early when they will stay down and work.

Drugs for motion sickness are listed in the Medical Equipment section (see page 97). All such medications cause drowsiness. Hyoscine is an anticholinergic drug that can be taken as a tablet or applied as a dermal patch behind the ear. Wash the hands after applying the patch so that hyoscine is not absorbed from them. A number of antihistamine preparations such as cyclizine and meclizine are helpful. Cinnarizine is popular in Europe and other countries outside the USA because of the balance between efficacious treatment and side effects.

Beware overdosing on anti-sickness medication. This can lead to tachycardia (fast pulse), dilated pupils (causing blurred vision), tremor, agitation and confusion.

Some crew on passage will become sick. A good skipper will spot the early signs and advise prompt action.

Anecdotal evidence suggests that the skipper and helmsman are less susceptible to sickness than other crew with no specific task. At the first sign of seasickness, one tactic is to give the sufferer the helm. This requires concentration but also allows the eyes to focus on the horizon.

Sick crew can sit in the cockpit wearing a harness and tether looking at the horizon. Once beyond any task they should move below and be placed in a comfortable warm bunk secured by a lee cloth with adequate supporting cushions (and a bucket). A completely empty stomach can render sickness worse. Loss of fluid from vomiting and the inability to take fluids will lead to dehydration and lethargy.

Isotonic drinks are preferable to water as they replace lost sodium. Oral medication is less helpful at this stage as tablets may not stay down. Hyoscine is a faster acting anti-emetic than most and can be taken by chewing or sublingually (under the tongue). In extreme cases an injection may be required.

These measures are usually enough to allow improvement. Some poor souls, however careful and disciplined, suffer the misery of profound unremitting illness. They can slump into a desperate catatonic state of hypothermia, fatigue, dehydration and vomiting semi-coma. The only cure is to reach dry land. As Spike Milligan said, 'The only sure cure for seasickness is to sit under a tree.'

A skipper must consider carefully which drugs to take on the voyage and remember that all drugs have side effects. Crew should be responsible for bringing a supply of their own prescription medications. Drugs for motion sickness are dealt with in the section Seasickness (see page 7). Antibiotics are discussed in the section Infections (see page 60). Drugs for analgesia (pain relief) are essential on a boat but must be chosen carefully.

**Paracetamol** (acetaminophen in the USA) will provide adequate relief for low level pain. Non-steroidal anti-inflammatories (NSAIDS) such as **ibuprofen**, **diclofenac** or **naproxen** can be taken with paracetamol and the effect is synergistic; the pain relief achieved is stronger than either drug alone. NSAIDS should be used with caution in those with asthma or gastritis. In some cases to administer an NSAID drug can cause fatality in an asthmatic patient. These drugs also cause bleeding from the stomach and so should be avoided in those with gastritis or stomach ulcer. **Aspirin** is an alternative analgesic to NSAIDS but both should be avoided in people on blood thinners. Combining these non-opioid analgesics will cover most moderate pain.

**Codeine** is a mild opioid and a stronger analgesic, which again is more effective in combination with non-opioid analgesics, for example it is available together with paracetamol as Co-codamol. A minority of people derive no benefit from codeine, lacking the ability to metabolise it. Codeine causes constipation so prolonged use is not advisable.

**Tramadol** is an effective prescription-only opioid and less addictive than morphine. The skipper must decide whether to carry aboard **morphine** (a strong opioid and prescription only). For serious trauma it can be invaluable but storing morphine aboard can present problems. If it is planned to take opioids on the boat, be sure to discuss with the prescribing doctor and arrange a secure place on the boat.

### Painkillers

| Mild pain | Non-opioid analgesics |
|---|---|
| | • **Paracetamol** 1g, 4 times a day |
| | • If needed add NSAID (**ibuprofen** 400mg, 3 times a day; **diclofenac** 50mg, 3 times a day or 100mg **suppository** 1 time a day; or **naproxen** 500mg, 2 times a day) |
| | • Or: **aspirin** 300mg, 4 times a day (maximum 4g a day) |
| Moderate pain | Mild opioid analgesics |
| | • **Codeine phosphate** 30mg, 4 times a day (can be combined with paracetamol as **co-codamol**) |
| | • Or: **tramadol** 50mg, 4 times a day |
| | • Plus: non-opioid analgesics |
| Severe pain | Strong opioid analgesics (stop weaker opioids but beware of respiratory depression) |
| | • **Morphine** 10mg or 20mg, 1 an hour; or **oxycodone** 5–10mg, 2 an hour |
| | • Plus: non-opioid analgesics |

If the patient cannot keep down the medication, perhaps through seasickness, then a different route of administration is required. Prescription-only opioids such as **fentanyl** can be taken sublingually (under the tongue) and tramadol can be administered as oral drops. Suppository is another mode for giving a drug. A suppository of diclofenac is a powerful painkiller. Injection is the most effective way of administering analgesia but requires needles and syringes and a degree of expertise. Such injections are best given intramuscularly into the front or outer aspect of the thigh. **Intravenous injections should only be given by those with the relevant skills.**

Drugs for acute medical emergencies such as anaphylaxis also present a problem. **Adrenaline**, present in the EpiPen, is dangerous if not used properly. Accidental administration can lead to cardiac problems and if injected in an inappropriate place, such as into the hand, can cause arterial spasm and even the loss of a finger. It is preferable to inject EpiPen only once and into the thigh.

Corticosteroids such as **prednisolone** can be helpful in the management of respiratory disease and allergy. A bottle of oxygen, say 400 litres, takes up storage space but may be live-saving for respiratory distress or collapse.

Other medications (such as antihistamines, hydrocortisone cream, antacids, laxatives and rehydration tablets) are covered in the appropriate chapters and listed in Medical Equipment under Drugs (see page 96).

Basic life support and cardiopulmonary resuscitation (CPR) should be started on any person who is unresponsive with abnormal or absent breathing (see the Basic Life Support table, page 19). It is not always easy to ascertain if someone is dead (has suffered a cardiac arrest), particularly if they have profound hypothermia. Assess if they are responsive by gently shaking and speaking loudly. If in doubt, resuscitation must be instituted.

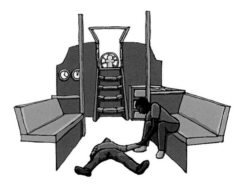

Move the patient to a place in the boat where resuscitation can most easily be performed. The cabin sole is the best place. It provides a firm base low in the vessel protected from the weather. As the patient is being moved to a suitable place, shout for help (if within range ask a crew member to call the Coast Guard or else an MRCC such as at Falmouth). Start with a rapid assessment using A, B, C – Airway, Breathing, Circulation.

**1** With the patient on their back, open the airway by tilting the head back.

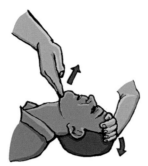

**2** Place one hand on the forehead, applying pressure to tilt the head back.

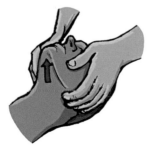

**3** Place fingers of the other hand under the chin and gently lift upward. Placing fingers under the angle of the jaw and lifting forwards (a jaw thrust) is also effective but takes two hands.

RESUSCITATION

**Airway**

If there is a suspicion of traumatic cervical spine injury, keep the head and neck as still as possible using manual in-line stabilisation: kneel behind the patient's head and place one hand either side of the head to minimise movement. If you are solo this will not be possible and you will have to prioritise resuscitation.

**4** Remove any foreign bodies that might obstruct breathing such as tongue, dentures, food, vomit and blood.

## Breathing

Take up to 10 seconds to check for breathing. Look for chest movement, listen at the patient's mouth for breathing, and feel for breath on your cheek. These three actions (looking, listening and feeling) can all be done simultaneously.

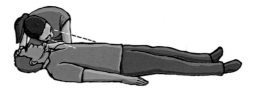

If the patient is breathing then place in the recovery position. If breathing is abnormal or absent start chest compressions.

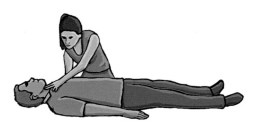

If there is any doubt over signs of life or a pulse, start CPR – do not delay. Time can be wasted seeking a pulse in a shocked or hypothermic patient. If you are trained, feel for a carotid pulse. (To become proficient at finding a pulse, practice gently on yourself or a friend at home but only try on one side of the neck at a time.)

## Chest compressions

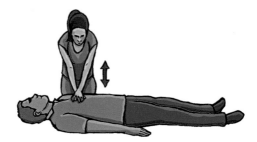

**1** To perform chest compressions effectively, lay the patient on a hard surface such as the cabin sole.

**2** Place the heel of one hand over the centre of the lower half of the sternum (breastbone), put the other hand on top and interlace the fingers.

**3** With the arms locked straight compress the chest by 5cm, or one third of the chest depth, at a rate of 100–120 compressions a minute – nearly twice every second.

Allow the chest to re-expand between each compression. Keep your hands in contact with the sternum, do not 'bounce' on the chest. For a child use only one hand.

## Rescue breathing

A rescue breath supplies oxygen to the lungs. If you are trained to perform rescue breaths, deliver 2 rescue breaths after 30 chest compressions.

**1** Kneel next to the patient's head.

**2** Be sure to maintain the open airway by tilting the head backwards.

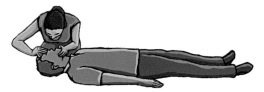

**3** Pinch the nostrils closed, take a breath, seal your lips around the mouth and blow.

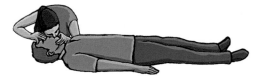

**4** Observe chest expansion then break the seal by removing your mouth and watch the chest exhale.

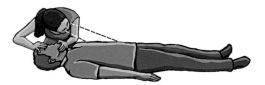

### Rescue breathing

If you are unable or unwilling to give rescue breaths, give continuous chest compressions. Properly administered chest compressions, without rescue breaths, can provide effective resuscitation.

---

**AT A GLANCE – Basic Life Support**
**Unresponsive and not breathing normally?**

◆ Call for help
◆ Attach AED if available
◆ 30 chest compressions
◆ 2 rescue breaths
◆ Continue CPR using 30:2 ratio

---

# Cardiopulmonary Resuscitation (CPR)

Call for help from the rest of the crew and begin CPR without delay. CPR is a combination of chest compressions and rescue breaths. **Perform rescue breaths at a rate of 2 breaths every 30 compressions.**

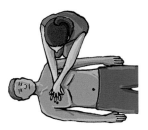

CPR can be exhausting and is best done by two or more people. The roles can be reversed and shared. Chest compressions alone are effective and can be continued without rescue breaths.

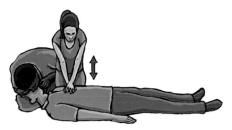

Minimise any interruptions to CPR and do not waste time by pausing to search for a pulse. CPR should be continued until breathing starts or the patient is considered beyond saving; persist for at least 30 minutes and in some cases

### Cardiopulmonary Resuscitation (CPR)

longer. CPR should be prolonged in cases of hypothermia, drowning, electrocution and in children, when you should continue for an hour if you are able.

If an Automated External Defibrillator (AED) is carried aboard it should be attached, turned on and the instructions followed as soon as possible after cardiac arrest is identified. In certain abnormal cardiac rhythms, ventricular fibrillation or pulseless ventricular tachycardia, a shock is necessary. For this reason some vessels carry an AED, which reads the heart rhythm and can be used by an untrained person. An AED is little use in remote areas – it is only worthwhile carrying one if evacuation to a medical facility can be arranged expeditiously.

**Early evacuation.** Patients who recover following CPR require early evacuation.

## Recovery position

A person with decreased consciousness who does not require CPR should be placed on their side in the recovery position.

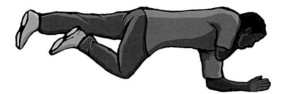

**1** Kneel beside the patient.

**2** Bend the arm closest to you at a right angle with palm up.

**3** Bring the far arm across the chest and rest the back of the hand on the cheek.

**4** Grasp the far leg behind the knee and bend the knee to a right angle.

**5** Keeping the hand against the cheek, pull on the far leg to roll the person towards you until they rest on their side.

**6** Tilt the head back to maintain an open airway. Check regularly for normal breathing.

## Choking

### *What to do about choking*

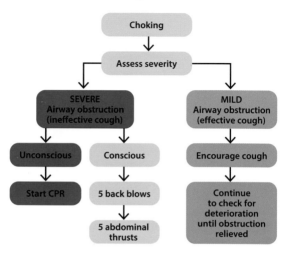

A foreign body can obstruct the airway and cause choking. The most common in fit people is a food, usually meat. Blood and vomit can also be to blame. If the obstruction is mild encourage the patient to cough. If the obstruction is severe (they are unable to speak or cough) give 5 back blows.

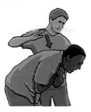

**1** Lean the patient forwards over an arm supporting the chest and give five firm and sharp blows on the back between the shoulder blades.

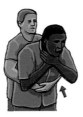

**2** If these back blows fail to relieve the obstruction then attempt abdominal thrusts.

**3** Stand behind the patient and put both arms around the upper part of the abdomen.

**4** Place one clenched fist in the upper abdomen below the sternum (breastbone), grab the fist with the other hand and pull sharply inwards and upwards. Repeat this up to 5 times.

It is wise to warn the patient before attempting these manoeuvres. If the patient becomes unconscious, start CPR, which may help in dislodging any foreign body.

## Unconscious crew

A crew member may collapse and become unconscious for various reasons. An unconscious person who is still breathing and has a pulse should be placed in the recovery position while the cause is established.

### *Causes of decreased consciousness*

| | |
|---|---|
| Trauma | ◆ Head injury |
| | ◆ Severe blood loss |
| | ◆ Drowning |
| | ◆ Electrocution |
| Syncope | Fainting due to: |
| | ◆ Low blood pressure |
| | ◆ Low blood sugar |
| | ◆ Dehydration |
| Allergy | Anaphylaxis due to food or an insect sting |
| Illness | ◆ Diabetes (low or high blood sugar) |
| | ◆ Heart attack |
| | ◆ Arrhythmia |
| | ◆ Stroke |
| | ◆ Epilepsy (seizure) |
| | ◆ Sepsis (severe infection) |
| Poisoning | ◆ Carbon monoxide |
| | ◆ Smoke inhalation |
| | ◆ Alcohol |
| | ◆ Drug overdose |

If the patient remains unconscious over a period of time beware of the pressure areas. Hips, knees, elbows and eyes are at particular risk. Use cushioning over pressure areas and be prepared to roll the patient every 2 hours or so. Secure them safely in a bunk with a lee cloth. If loss of consciousness has lasted more than 2 hours consider catheterising the bladder (a boat sailing any distance offshore should carry a catheter).

### *A, B, C*

| | |
|---|---|
| Airway | Check airway is open and unobstructed |
| Breathing | Check the patient is breathing |
| Circulation | Check the heart is pumping by feeling the carotid pulse |

**Early evacuation.** An unconscious patient requires early evacuation.

## Minor wounds: cuts and lacerations

Cuts are caused by sharp edges while a laceration is more of a tear to the skin. They should be inspected for foreign material such as wood splinters or grease and then washed with antiseptic. A clean cut can be closed by suture, staple, tape or glue and covered with a sterile dressing.

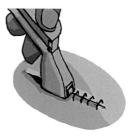

Although wound tapes are the easiest to apply, they are not suitable if the skin is wet or over a joint that may be flexed. If using glue, care must be taken to prevent spillage onto other parts of the patient or onto the carer (don't glue yourself to the patient). Glue should only be used on straight, dry, non-bleeding wounds and not used for cuts over joints.

Suturing and stapling require a level of expertise that is easily attained on a first aid course. Staples when properly applied have the advantage of speed but do not use them on the face. Suturing will stop skin edge bleeding, which in the case of the scalp can be profuse.

A dirty, contaminated cut or ragged laceration should be cleansed, foreign material removed, thoroughly rinsed in antiseptic solution and left unsutured and open before a sterile dressing is applied. If antiseptic solution is unavailable or has run out, then use boiled (and then cooled) salt water.

Hands can be injured by fishhooks, knives, scalding, rope burns and more. Even minor hand injuries must be taken seriously. It is difficult to help run a boat with only one functioning hand.

On deck, bare feet are susceptible to injury and below deck from scalding in the galley. Very severe injuries to hands or feet, even with the loss of a digit, can be inflicted by the anchor windlass, electric winches, engine, prop shaft, propeller and in the galley.

### Fishhook injuries
Remove a fishhook by pushing it on through, by removing the barb or by the string technique.

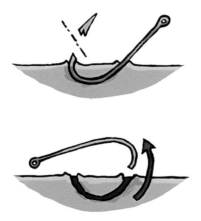

The injured hand must be washed with antiseptic and dressed with a non-stick dressing. Keep the fingers apart by dressing them separately. The fingernail may be partially avulsed. This is a painful injury that can bleed. Do not try to remove the nail. Instead replace it into position and cover with a soft dressing held in place with a bandage.

### *Fingernail injuries*

A painful haematoma or bruise may occur under the nail following crushing or a heavy blow to the finger. The nail will appear black and be extremely painful. The haematoma should be released. This is best achieved by burning a hole through the nail with a hot pin or paperclip heated in a flame and held with pliers. Continue applying the pin until loss of resistance is felt and the blood escapes. This procedure is surprisingly pain free.

### *Crush injuries*

Crushing injury of the hand or foot can damage deep tissues such as muscles and tendons and bone as well as the skin. A crush injury causes extremely painful and intense swelling even though bleeding may be slight. Elevate and cool the limb to reduce swelling. Once the swelling eases, the pain will recede but meanwhile give adequate pain relief.

**Early evacuation.** A severe hand injury with loss of function requires early evacuation.

Bleeding is best staunched by direct pressure over the bleeding point with a sterile dressing for at least 10 minutes.

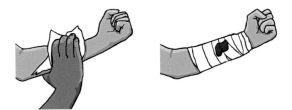

- Bandage the bleeding point firmly.
- If a limb is bleeding, lay the patient down, apply the bandage and elevate the part.
- If blood appears through the bandage, then apply another dressing and a second firm bandage over the first. Do not remove the initial dressing as this may disturb blood clotting.
- Be sure not to bandage so tightly that the circulation to the extremity is compromised.
- Analgesia (pain relief) may be required as pain can make shock worse.
- Fluids to replace the loss of blood should be administered.
- Care must be exercised when pressing directly near the trachea (windpipe) or the eye.

### *Tourniquets*

Unless you are experienced do not apply a makeshift tourniquet. Injudicious application of a tourniquet, by obstructing the veins but failing properly to occlude the arteries, can exacerbate haemorrhage from a limb. A tight tourniquet will cut off the circulation to the limb. Only attempt to apply a tourniquet if haemorrhage from the limb is life-threatening.

If a tourniquet is to be applied, it should be at least 5 cm wide and flat so that it does not cut through the skin. A wide sail tie placed over a bandage to protect the skin will do.

**1** Pass the tourniquet around the limb and tie a knot.
**2** Put a stick or metal rod on the knot and tie another knot over the rod. Then twist the rod as a Spanish windlass to tighten the tourniquet.

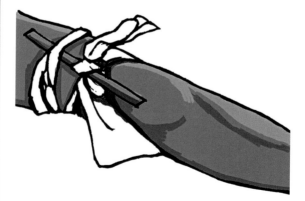

**3** Tie the other end of the rod to prevent it unwinding.

**4** Note the time when the tourniquet was applied. After an hour gently loosen the tourniquet to allow blood to the extremity. Bleeding may have eased sufficiently for it to be controlled by direct pressure. If not then twist the Spanish windlass again.

---

*AT A GLANCE – Bleeding*
- Staunch the bleeding by direct pressure
- Apply sterile dressing and firm bandage
- Elevate the bleeding body part

---

**Early evacuation.** A patient suffering major haemorrhage that cannot be adequately staunched requires early evacuation.

## Fractures

A fracture at sea is always serious and if it involves a long bone extremely serious. Any kind of fracture can be painful and difficult to treat and leaves the rest of the boat's crew short-handed. Fractures of large bones such as the pelvis or femur may be associated with significant blood loss. Intense swelling or the acutely angled leg bones can obstruct the circulation in the limb.

In principle fractures should be gently reduced (by pulling, straightening and putting the bone back in line) and then immobilised with a splint.

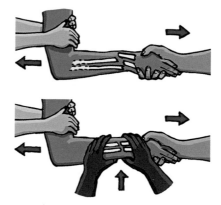

Immobilisation is crucial as it is movement of the fracture that causes severe pain. Analgesia and fluids, the treatment of shock, are important in the management of a fracture. The patient with a broken bone, especially a break of the leg, needs to be immobilised in a bunk with a lee cloth to prevent further injury.

### *Compound fractures*

A compound fracture is one where the skin is broken. The bone may or may not be protruding from the wound. Such a fracture makes things more complicated because of the risk of infection and for that reason should be cleaned with antiseptic solution.

---

**AT A GLANCE – Fractures**

- ◆ Reduce the fracture and re-align the bones
- ◆ Immobilise the fracture with a splint or sling
- ◆ Immobilise the patient in a bunk to avoid further injury
- ◆ Give pain relief
- ◆ Give fluids
- ◆ Give antibiotics if fracture is compound

---

**TRAUMA AND INJURIES**

## Specific fractures

### Finger or toe fracture/dislocation

The fracture/dislocation should be reduced as quickly as possible by pulling the digit before sensation returns. The injured digit, usually a finger, should then be strapped to an adjoining finger or a finger splint.

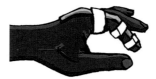

A dislocation should be immobilised in this way for a week or so, a fracture for several weeks.

### Forearm and wrist (radius and ulna)

Reduce the fracture by gently pulling and straightening then, if possible, apply a splint from above the elbow, bent to a right angle, to the hand. Curl the hand and fingers around something soft like a length of rolled-up bandage.

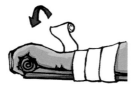 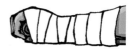

### *Upper arm (humerus)*

Use a bandage to make a collar and cuff. Support the arm by tying the bandage around the wrist and up around the neck.

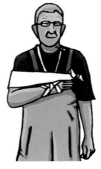

The weight of the arm will help to reduce the fracture. A second broad bandage can hold the arm to the side.

### *Clavicle*

Support the arm in a sling.

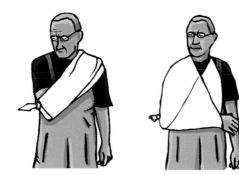

### *Upper leg (femur)*

The other leg can be used as a splint. Place soft padding between the legs – a pillow works well. In addition and for extra effective splinting, a storm board or oar with plenty of padding can be strapped down the outside of the leg.

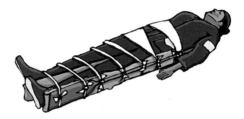

The splint should immobilise the joint above and below the fracture. This means that the outer splint must reach at least as high as the abdomen or chest.

### *Lower leg (tibia)*

Place a pillow between the legs and a padded outer splint up to thigh, level high enough to immobilise the knee.

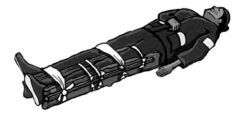

### Ankle

Distinguishing between a fracture, dislocation or sprain can be difficult. For any of these, immobilise the foot in the neutral position with the ankle at a right angle. A U-shaped splint may help. Elevate the foot.

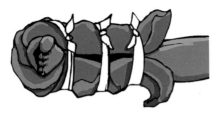

### Jaw

A fracture of the jaw causes pain in the face and jaw, mainly located in front of the ear on the affected side, and worse on movement. The face will be swollen and bruised and blood may ooze from the mouth. The patient will have difficulty opening or closing their mouth. Remove broken teeth and blood. Lean the patient forwards to allow blood and fluids to drain. Maintain their airway at all costs. Apply a Barton head bandage.

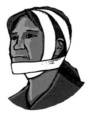

Commence antiseptic mouth washes and start antibiotics. Allow only fluids by mouth.

## Specific fractures

### *Ribs*

Sit the patient upright. They may need to be comfortably wedged in position against the roll of the boat. Multiple rib fractures may cause difficulty with breathing and reduce the amount of oxygen reaching the lungs. Give plenty of analgesia but do not give opiates, which can depress breathing. Specific measures such a strapping are not usually helpful. Should there be an open sucking wound immediately cover it, initially with a hand, then apply a sterile or clean dressing to seal the wound and render it airtight.

**Early evacuation.** A patient with a fracture of pelvis, upper leg, jaw or multiple ribs requires early evacuation.

Minor head injuries at sea are common. Children now wear helmets when sailing dinghies. More adults also wear helmets sailing yachts, especially at the start of a race when manoeuvring briskly.

A severe head injury from the boom can be fatal. In a gybe, for instance, as the boom swings across, either the boom or the mainsheet can cause severe, even lethal, damage. More than ever in this situation prevention is better than cure – avoid a head injury at all costs. Employ a boom preventer or a boom brake. When sailing downwind in heavy weather consider dropping the main, fixing the boom and running on headsails alone. When going over the side to inspect the hull or propeller or when climbing the mast, wear a helmet. A simple climber's helmet will suffice.

Concussion is a short period of unconsciousness or confusion followed by rapid recovery. There may be amnesia of the event. Pain in the injured area may be eased and the swelling reduced by holding a cold compress, such as a bag of ice cubes, to it intermittently for short periods. Associated headaches can be treated with analgesia such as paracetamol.

The patient should be carefully monitored for deterioration. Later symptoms may include continued headache, drowsiness, nausea, vomiting, double vision, confusion, fitting and further loss of consciousness. Such deterioration is extremely serious and early evacuation must be considered.

In the case of severe head injury when the patient is unconscious with no recovery, open the airway, immobilise the cervical spine perhaps with a collar and place in a bunk with supporting pillows. Check for other injuries. Bleeding, for instance from a scalp wound, should be staunched by direct pressure and later suture.

## Head injuries

The unconscious patient must be monitored and have the pulse rate, breathing rate, pupil size and response recorded every half hour. For response, record the conscious level (AVPU – see the table below) and the times. This will provide a sufficient record at sea. The Glasgow Coma Scale (GCS) is another, more detailed, method of recording level of consciousness using eye, motor and verbal responses. The important point in the case of an unconscious patient is to record carefully the responses and the times.

### *Monitor consciousness level: A, V, P, U*

| A | Alert | Alert |
|---|-------|-------|
| V | Vocal | Response to vocal stimuli, by speech or eye opening |
| P | Pain | Response to painful stimuli by speech, eye opening or movement |
| U | Unresponsive | Unresponsive to any stimulus |

### *AT A GLANCE – Head injuries*
◆ Open the airway
◆ Immobilise neck
◆ Check for other injuries
◆ Place in recovery position (if cervical spine intact)
◆ Monitor conscious level (AVPU)

**Early evacuation.** A patient who remains unconscious from head injury requires early evacuation.

Burns can be life-threatening. Patients with significant burns can suffer severe pain, fluid loss sufficient to cause renal failure, infection leading to sepsis and smoke inhalation.

Common causes of fire aboard are burning fat or scalding water in the galley, fuel on a hot exhaust and an electrical fault. An electrical burn is always full thickness and often the damage is more extensive than appears at first glance. Burns from chemicals or the sun can become serious too.

To avoid such events wear an apron and shoes when cooking in the galley or on a barbecue. In rough weather avoid boiling water, use pots with lids such as a pressure cooker or, even safer, employ the oven.

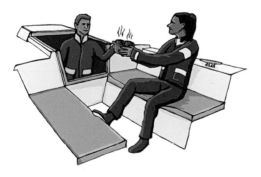

Do not pass hot cups of soup or tea by hand but in a receptacle such as a washing up bowl. Do not work on a hot engine. In the sun, wear a hat, shirt and sunblock.

### *Initial treatment*

**1** Move the patient away from the source of the heat. If the clothes are on fire then smother the flames with a blanket or 'drop and roll' (this is less easy at sea).

**2** Remove any non-adherent clothing and jewellery near to the burn.

**3** Remove heat from the area by cooling.

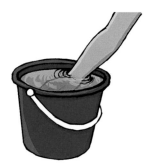

This is best done with cold water but not ice. A burnt extremity should be plunged into cold water for 20 minutes or more. This action removes heat, excludes air and offers some pain relief. A large quantity of water may be required so, on the ocean, this may mean using seawater.

If the torso or trunk is burnt and plunging into water is not possible then use wet towels and refresh the cold water frequently. A chemical burn must be flushed with water for at least 15 minutes.

**4** Cover the burn to reduce the amount of fluid loss and the chance of contamination leading to subsequent infection.

This is best done with a hydrogel burns dressing that will cool the burnt skin, thus reducing pain, and provide a sterile dressing that conforms to the contours of the body. If such dressings are not available use clingfilm. Lay it on the burn and lightly apply a bandage to hold it in place.

If a hand is burnt or scalded, wrap each finger individually with dressing or clingfilm to prevent them sticking together and place the whole hand in a clean plastic bag.

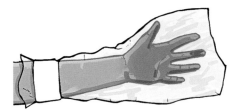

Do not apply any creams, oils or butter. Blisters should be left intact as they act in the same way as a dressing, keeping out air and helping to prevent infection.

### *Later assessment*

After 48 hours check for signs of infection such as increased pain, odour, excessive exudate (pus), redness or fever. Change the dressing if needed. If it is dry and comfortable leave undisturbed for 5 days. Thereafter change the dressing every 3 to 5 days until the wound is healed.

The depth of a burn may be described as superficial, partial thickness or full thickness. **Superficial burns** give rise to reddened skin and are painful and tender to touch. With appropriate treatment subsequent scarring is absent or minimal. With a **partial thickness burn** the skin is red and blistered and extremely painful and tender.

A **full thickness burn** can exhibit leathery, sometimes blackened skin. The skin and underlying tissue such as muscle and tendon may be charred. The full thickness burn is not painful as the nerve endings have been destroyed. However, the area of skin around the burn can be very painful. Partial and full thickness burns heal but with debilitating scarring and contractures.

### *The Rule of Nines*
The area of a burn can be estimated by the Rule of Nines.

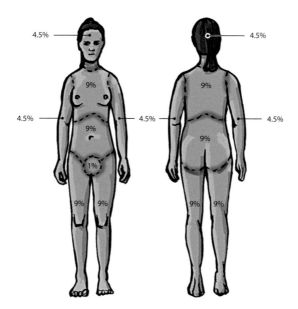

4.5%     4.5%

9%     9%

4.5%     4.5%     4.5%

9%     9%

1%

9%     9%     9%     9%

Each region of the body as illustrated is equivalent to 9% of the body surface area. The palm is equivalent to 1% surface area and the area of an open hand with fingers splayed around 4%. These figures will help the skipper estimate the body surface area burnt.

### *Smoke inhalation*
Smoke inhalation can be serious. It may be suspected if the patient has a reddened, blistered face, burnt eyebrows or soot at the back of the mouth. Symptoms include hoarse voice with rapid, difficult, noisy breathing. The patient may initially appear well before later deterioration. Sit the patient upright as the lungs work more efficiently in this position. Administer oxygen if you have any.

---

**AT A GLANCE – Burns**
- ◆ Remove from source of heat
- ◆ Cool the burn
- ◆ Dress the burn
- ◆ Give pain relief
- ◆ Give fluids
- ◆ Give antibiotics if infected

---

**Early evacuation.** Patients who suffer burns to the face, hands or genitals, deep burns or those covering more than 5% body surface area or significant symptoms of smoke inhalation require early evacuation. So do all children who suffer burns.

## Hypothermia and drowning

### Hypothermia

Hypothermia does not require immersion. It can occur after a prolonged period on deck. Symptoms include irritability, lethargy, slurred speech, loss of memory and eventually an unresponsive state leading to coma.

The sufferer must be brought below deck for warming. Wrap the patient in warm covers and a foil blanket and lie them in a bunk in the recovery position. Someone should lie down alongside to help the warming process. If the patient is conscious offer a hot sweet drink.

### Drowning

The possibility of drowning is a risk for all those who go to sea. People who are drowning do not cry out or wave. In the brief time the mouth is above the water, the need to breathe takes priority over yelling. If they raise their arms to wave they sink further, so they don't. It has been estimated that in 10% of cases when children drown, an adult will actually watch them drown having no idea it is happening.

With drowning, just as with head injury, prevention is of paramount importance as treatment is not always successful in the event of either. Prevention is simple: wear a life jacket and fasten the crotch strap. This applies to everyone on the water, paddleboarders, kayakers, dinghy sailors, motor boaters, yachtsmen. Of those people who drown not wearing a life jacket, it is thought that around 85% would have survived if they had been wearing one.

Sailors should wear a life jacket, harness and tether when sailing at night, in heavy weather (even when resting below), working forward of the mast, when alone on deck and when performing a tricky manoeuvre such as shortening sail. It is wise, and indeed law in some countries, to wear a lifejacket in a dinghy. The return trip in the dark from a meal ashore represents a risk and crew have drowned in that short trip. The modern life jacket is so light and easy to wear there is an argument to wear one all the time when aboard.

## What to do about drowning

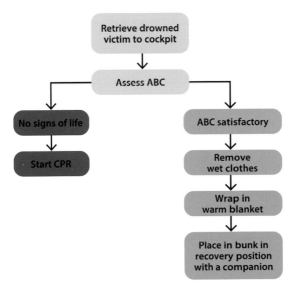

**TRAUMA AND INJURIES**

## Treatment

1 Once the drowned patient has been hauled back aboard or to the shore, assess them for signs of life and check for A, B and C: Airway, Breathing and Circulation (see page 13).

2 If these are satisfactory then roll the patient into the recovery position. There is no purpose in performing the Heimlich manoeuvre or abdominal thrusts to empty the lungs – if the patient is alive the volume of water in the lungs will be quite small.

3 It is essential to remove wet clothing and then to wrap the patient in warm covers; continue treatment as for hypothermia.

4 If there is no sign of life then begin CPR with chest compressions following Basic Life Support guidance (see page 19). For cases of hypothermia and drowning CPR should be continued for an hour, especially in children.

**Early evacuation.** A patient resuscitated from cardiac arrest from hypothermia or drowning requires early evacuation.

### *Eye injuries*

The eye is well protected within the bony orbit and eye injuries are rare. However, they can be caused by a flogging rope such as a jib sheet or a flapping sail, for example. If an injury is suspected because of pain and/or streaming tears then examine the eye. Observe the pupil size compared to the other eye.

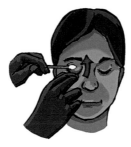

Gently pull down the lower eyelid and evert the upper eyelid. This may reveal a foreign body, red sclera, blood in the eye behind the cornea and in front of the iris.

Extreme pain in the eye associated with a sensation of a foreign body in the eye may suggest a corneal abrasion. It will not be possible to see this at sea even with a magnifying glass. A corneal abrasion will usually heal within a few days. A penetrating eye injury may not always be obvious. If a fishhook is caught in the eye, do not attempt to remove it, but ensure early evacuation with the patient.

### Treatment

- Remove any foreign body that has not penetrated the eye.
- A corneal abrasion is extremely painful and this can be relieved by giving local anaesthetic eye drops inside the lower eyelid.

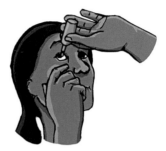

- If the eye has been affected by a chemical thoroughly wash the eye with water, preferably sterile, or with saline for at least 15 minutes. If the chemical was alkali then wash for longer.
- In all cases of trauma or chemical injury, the eye should be treated with chloramphenicol antibiotic drops or ointment to prevent infection; the latter lasts longer. In severe cases, such as a penetrating injury, administer oral antibiotics as well.
- Eye injuries are painful so analgesia, including local anaesthetic eye drops and oral painkillers, should be given.

### Eye disorders

**Contact lenses** can cause problems at sea. Wearers may suffer dry eyes, conjunctivitis and corneal abrasion. The treatment is to stop wearing the lenses and give artificial tears or chloramphenicol ointment. A lens can be lost under an eyelid and must be retrieved – most wearers will have had to do this before and will know how.

**Sea blindness** is similar to mountaineer's snow blindness. It is caused by damage to the cornea from UV rays. Patients suffer extreme pain in the eye and photophobia. Prevention by wearing good quality sunglasses is best. Otherwise administer local anaesthetic drops and antibiotic ointment.

A bright red **subconjunctival haemorrhage** looks alarming but is painless and does not affect vision. No specific treatment is needed. So called 'red eye' can be serious, especially if painful, and may be due to acute glaucoma, acute iritis, or orbital cellulitis (infection).

**Early evacuation.** A penetrating eye injury, a painful red eye without trauma and acute blindness require early evacuation.

## Ears

Outer ear infection or otitis externa, sometimes called **swimmer's ear**, is the most likely affliction to occur on a boat. It appears as a painful ear with discharge, sometimes with pus. Pulling the earlobe is painful. Avoid further swimming. Rinse the ear with sterile water or vinegar. If symptoms persist, use antibiotic ear drops at the rate of 4 drops into the ear every 6 hours for up to a week. Chloramphenicol eye ointment or drops may be used if specific ear drops are unavailable.

To have a buzzing insect trapped in the ear is extremely distressing; it drives people crazy. Treat it by administering a few drops of olive oil into the ear. This will cause the death of the insect. Then remove the corpse carefully with tweezers.

A **nosebleed** can be alarming. The majority come from the anterior (front) part of the nose and respond well to simple treatment. A bleed from the back of the nose is more difficult to treat. The blood may be bright red, which signifies active bleeding or dark with clots.

### Treatment
1 Sit the patient upright or, if they are unable to do this comfortably, in a reclining position.
2 Squeeze the anterior, soft, part of the nose between index finger and thumb for at least 15 minutes, the patient may be able to do this themselves.
3 This will usually control the bleeding but if it continues then repeat the manoeuvre for another 20 minutes.

If the bleeding continues even when the nose is being pinched, it indicates a bleed from the posterior or back part of the nasal cavity. If it fails to abate, then packing the nose may be necessary.

1 Cut a strip of clean cotton cloth, up to a metre may be needed. Cover the strip with petroleum jelly (Vaseline) or an antibiotic ointment.
2 Pack it gently into the nose, starting at the middle of the strip so that, when packed, both ends protrude from the nostril. Use tweezers and a piece of wood such as a fine chopstick or a twig. Alternatively pack the nose with a tampon.
3 The nose contains bacteria so give antibiotics (amoxycillin or azithromycin) until the pack is removed.
4 Leave the pack or tampon in situ for one or two days.
5 If bleeding recommences, gently blow the nose to remove clots and then repack.

### Nose

Another more specialist approach to stop the bleeding from the back of the nose is to use a urinary catheter. One should be in the medical kit for treating acute retention of urine. The Foley type catheter should be introduced into the nose as far as the back of the throat. The tip will be visible through the open mouth. Inject into the balloon 10 or 15ml of air and gently withdraw the catheter through the nose until it impacts upon and obstructs the bleeding area.

The deformity of a **broken nose** may be obvious after facial trauma. It is sometimes possible immediately to grab the nose and straighten it. If this painful procedure proves unsuccessful then do not persist, leave it until proper treatment can be given ashore. A broken nose alone or a nosebleed are rarely reasons for early evacuation.

Visit a dentist before setting out on a long voyage. In the medical kit include a dental mirror, tweezers, a first aid dental kit such as Dentanurse and a temporary filling material like Cavit.

**Toothache** without infection is usually caused by a cavity (a hole in the enamel). The treatment is to dry the hole and apply oil of cloves (eugenol) then fill the hole using a temporary filling material. Semi-melted candle wax can suffice.

A **tooth abscess** gives rise to an intense throbbing pain and tenderness, sometimes with swelling of the face or neck. Antibiotics must be given (metronidazole and co-amoxiclav). That may be enough but if the pain is associated with an old filling, remove what you can and clean the resultant hole with antiseptic. Leave the hole to drain.

If a **tooth is knocked out** by facial trauma, it should be replaced in under an hour so that it may survive. Handle the tooth by the crown. Gently rinse the root but do not abrade it. To keep the tooth, perhaps for another attempt to implant it, store it in a container with milk. Should the tooth socket continue to bleed, roll up a piece of gauze, place it in the empty socket and ask the patient to bite on it for 20 minutes or so.

## Skin

It is important for everyone on board take care to protect their skin.

### Sunburn

Sunburn can become quite debilitating so protective measures must be taken. Do not rely entirely on sunblock, which can become diluted by sweat or washed away when swimming. Limit the time spent in glaring sun. In fierce sun, wear a long-sleeved shirt, a wide-brimmed hat and long trousers. Sunglasses will protect against glare and prevent sea blindness (sunburn of the cornea and similar to snow blindness). If a person becomes severely sunburnt move them into the shade and give fluids to maintain hydration. Apply a cold compress to the affected area. If needed give pain relief such as paracetamol together with an NSAID such as ibuprofen. Calamine lotion may sooth sunburnt skin. In severe cases hydrocortisone 1% cream may help.

### Rashes

Skin rashes may be due to infection, allergic reactions or inflammation. An allergic rash is red and sometimes urticarial, meaning that the skin is raised and swollen (also called hives). The common causes on a boat are drugs and chemicals. Remove the probable cause and stop any suspected drug. Antihistamines will help either applied to the skin (diphenhydramine cream, such as Benadryl) or taken orally (chlorpheniramine tablets, such as Piriton).

### Impetigo

Impetigo is a staphylococcal skin infection. It starts with small, infected blisters that become pustular, break down into running sores and leave crusty patches (like corn flakes on the skin). To treat, clean the affected skin with antiseptic solution, dry the area and apply antibiotic cream. If infection is extensive also give oral antibiotics such as flucloxacillin effective against staphylococci or, if penicillin allergic, clarithromycin.

### Eczema

Eczema (dermatitis) is a common, chronic condition and the patient is usually aware of the diagnosis. Patches of skin become red and scaly. If the patch is wet attempt to dry it and if dry then use moisturiser. In acute severe cases hydrocortisone 1% cream will help.

### Shingles

Shingles causes an area of skin on one side of the body to become painful. This pain is followed soon after by a vesicular (small blisters) rash. There is no specific treatment and the rash should settle in a week or two.

### Blisters

Blisters are best avoided and another example where prevention is better than cure. To protect the hands wear gloves when working the anchor, chain, ropes or helming in rough weather. Wearing shoes of some sort is wise as feet can be injured and blister when on deck or below.

At the first sign of chafing protect the part and cover with a blister dressing. A doughnut dressing can be constructed by cutting a hole in the dressing immediately over the part.

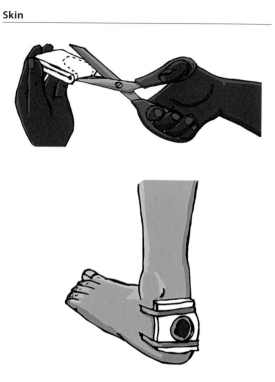

Small blisters are best left alone. Larger blisters can be pricked with a sterile needle and the fluid milked out. Leave the redundant skin and protect with a dressing, preferably a hydrogel burns dressing or hydrocolloid dressing.

# Frostbite

Frostbite signifies that the skin and maybe the deeper tissues are frozen. This is most likely to occur at high latitude but with careful attention can usually be avoided.

Frostbite occurs on the extremities, the hands, feet, nose, ears and, in bad cases, the cheeks. The skin will be white, sometimes with a purple hue. The affected part feels cold and hard like wood and will eventually blister.

## *Treatment*

- Protect the area from further cold and from trauma, and keep the patient warm, hydrated and fed.
- Administer a low dose of aspirin 75mg and ibuprofen 400mg three times daily. This medication will help the pain and the circulation.
- Smoking and alcohol should be avoided.
- Do not rub or massage the affected part – this will cause further trauma.
- To rewarm the extremity, such as a hand, place it in warm water of about 40°C (but not more than 43°C) with some antiseptic added. This may take an hour.
- When the hand has thawed, it will become red, throbbing, painful, swollen and blistered.
- If there is no prospect of early evacuation of the patient it may be necessary to repeat the above.

# Infections

Infections are caught more readily in port than at sea. They can be viral, bacterial, fungal and parasitic. Not all infections require antibiotics. Viral infections such as influenza, norovirus enteritis or coronavirus do not respond to antibiotic therapy.

Antibiotics may not be needed for an unclean open wound, abrasion or laceration. Such wounds should be cleansed with antiseptic solution, have any foreign material removed, cleansed with antiseptic again and kept dry. If the wound develops surrounding redness and swelling, indicative of infection, antibiotic therapy should be given.

If antibiotics are not available, supportive measures can help. Wounds, ears and eyes can be washed with boiled salt water (two cups of cooled boiled water with one teaspoon of salt and a pinch of baking soda). Abscesses can be soaked in warm saline or a poultice and encouraged to discharge pus. A person with a chest infection can sit up, energetically cough up phlegm, breathe deeply and take in a steam inhalant.

It is a good idea to take antibiotics on any offshore voyage. When deciding on an antibiotic, try to give the best one for the task. A **broad-spectrum antibiotic** such as ciprofloxacin will treat severe bacterial gastroenteritis, and co-amoxiclav will treat pneumonia or a urinary tract infection. A **penicillin** such as flucloxacillin or amoxicillin will treat skin infections. **Non-penicillin antibiotics** (clarithromycin, doxycycline) must be administered for those with penicillin allergy (see box). An antibiotic for anaerobic infection (metronidazole) is useful for targeting mouth infections and dental abscesses.

A more comprehensive list of antibiotics can be found in the table on page 96.

**Penicillin allergy** is a potential and dangerous problem and should always be ruled out where possible. The patient often knows of their allergy. In such cases use a non-penicillin alternative even if considered less efficacious.

Specific infections such as chest or urinary infections are tackled in their own sections of the book (see page 66 and 77).

### Antibiotics and antifungals

| BODY SYSTEM | INFECTION | DRUG (penicillins highlighted in bold – beware: may cause severe reaction in the allergic) |
|---|---|---|
| Abdomen | Bacterial gastroenteritis, bloody diarrhoea | Ciprofloxacin, Metronidazole |
| Chest | Pneumonia | **Amoxicillin**, **Co-amoxiclav**, Clarithromycin, Doxycycline |
| Ears | Otitis externa | Sofradex ear drops, Otomize ear spray, Ciprofloxacin |
| Eyes | Bacterial conjunctivitis | Chloramphenicol eye drops/ointment |
| Dental | Gingivitis, periodontitis, dental abscess | Metronidazole, Doxycyline, **Amoxicillin** |

ACUTE MEDICAL ILLNESS

| BODY SYSTEM | INFECTION | DRUG (penicillins highlighted in bold – beware: may cause severe reaction in the allergic) |
|---|---|---|
| Skin | Impetigo, cellulitis, wound infection, infected burn, Athlete's foot | **Amoxicillin**, **Flucloxacillin**, **Co-amoxiclav**, Clarithromycin, Co-trimoxazole 1% cream |
| Urine | Cystitis, pyelonephritis | **Co-amoxiclav**, Ciprofoxacin |
| Genital | Sexually transmitted infection, pelvic inflammation, vaginal thrush | Doxycycline, Co-trimoxazole 1% cream |

# Anaphylaxis

Anaphylaxis is a severe allergic reaction that can occur in response to an insect or jellyfish sting, drugs and some foods such as peanuts. The patient will notice itchy skin and eyes, a red rash, sweating, faintness from low blood pressure, shortness of breath and wheezy breathing, swelling of the lips, and constriction of the throat. This may be followed by complete collapse with respiratory or cardiac arrest.

## *Treatment*

The patient may have an EpiPen device that can administer adrenaline by intramuscular injection. It is worth considering keeping an EpiPen in the ship's medical kit. The usual dose is 0.5mg or 0.5 ml of 1:1,000 adrenaline solution. This may be repeated every 10 minutes but only if the patient is not responding. The intramuscular injection is best given in the front or side of the thigh. Timely administration of adrenaline is critical and lifesaving.

In addition an antihistamine such as chlorpheniramine 20mg and a steroid, either hydrocortisone 100mg or prednisolone 50mg, should be given although their onset of action is much slower than adrenaline. A salbutamol inhaler will help wheezing, give 4 puffs initially followed by 4 puffs every 5 minutes. Give oxygen if available. If complete collapse has occurred start CPR and administer adrenaline.

**Early evacuation.** A patient who has suffered an anaphylactic shock with collapse requires early evacuation.

## Diabetes

Diabetes is a condition characterised by inadequate production of insulin for the body's metabolic needs. The disease is becoming more common and the skipper must be informed if one of the crew is diabetic.

### Hypoglycaemia

Serious symptoms occur if the **blood sugar is too low** (hypoglycaemia), which can happen if more insulin or oral diabetic medication is taken than the food and sugar intake requires. A diabetic who suffers seasickness with loss of appetite and vomiting will have difficulty with their diabetic control and may become hypoglycaemic.

The patient may become sweaty, appear confused and aggressive like someone who is drunk, develop slurred speech and eventually lose consciousness. Should this happen when on watch and helming, the consequences for the boat will be serious, which is why the skipper must know of the condition. The treatment is to administer sugar with a sweet drink or a biscuit or similar.

### Hyperglycaemia

**High blood sugar** (hyperglycaemia) can also occur aboard a boat and is the result of too little insulin. The crew member may have omitted an insulin dose, perhaps due to feeling seasick and unwell. Symptoms include lethargy, continuous thirst, passing large amounts of urine, rapid breathing and eventually loss of consciousness. They will become dehydrated so give regular sips of water. If it is uncertain from the symptoms whether the patient has high or low blood sugar then it is safer to administer sugar.

### *Anti-diabetic drugs*

Familiarise yourself with a diabetic crew member's medication regimen as they can vary widely. Type 2 Diabetics may only require anti-diabetic drugs taken by mouth. Type 1 Diabetics or those with poorly controlled Type 2 diabetes require insulin. Types of insulin include rapid acting (Novorapid, Humalog), short acting (Actrapid, Humalin S), intermediate acting (Insulatard, Humalin I), long acting (insulin glargine) and mixed (Humalin Mix25). Insulin can be extremely dangerous if given without appropriate training so exercise caution if helping a sick diabetic to administer their insulin.

**Early evacuation.** An unconscious diabetic not responding to treatment requires early evacuation.

**ACUTE MEDICAL ILLNESS**

## Chest disorders

### *Asthma*

Unaccustomed exercise on a boat together with cold weather and forgetting regular use of inhalers can set off an asthma attack. Symptoms include shortness of breath and wheezing with a fast respiratory rate. The patient will be sitting up braced forwards. If they cannot complete a whole sentence then their condition is severe.

### Treatment

- Sit the person up and administer a bronchodilator, such as salbutamol inhaler. The person is likely to have their own inhaler.
- Give oxygen if available.
- A short course of a steroid such as prednisolone will help an exacerbation of asthma.
- **In extremis** when facing imminent respiratory arrest, inject adrenaline from an EpiPen. Such severe asthma usually occurs in children.

**Early evacuation.** Patients suffering from severe asthma, especially children, require early evacuation.

### *Chest infections*

Chest infections manifest with a fever, shortness of breath, a fast respiratory rate, cough, green sputum and maybe some wheezing. Pleurisy can complicate a chest infection and causes sharp pain when breathing in or coughing. The patient should be sat up to help their breathing and given antibiotics; amoxicillin is suitable, or doxycycline if penicillin allergic. If the infection is severe with a breathing rate of 40/min or more, give oxygen if available.

*Chest pains*

Angina is cardiac pain due to reduced blood flow to the heart muscle. The pain occurs on exertion but is absent at rest. Most sufferers will have glyceryl trinitrate (GTN) tablets that dissolve under the tongue. The question arises whether those with heart disease and angina should take the risk and sail any distance from shore.

The chest pain of a heart attack is severe – crushing in nature, felt in the central chest and can radiate into the jaw and down both arms, particularly the left arm. A heart attack can be accompanied by pallor, sweating, shortness of breath, faintness, nausea, anxiety and a sense of impending doom.

### Treatment

- To treat a heart attack give an aspirin (300mg tablet) immediately and a further half tablet daily if medical evacuation and further specialist treatment is not feasible.
- Pain relief is important and may require morphine by intramuscular injection. The patient may have GTN tablets or a nitroglycerin spray and these should be given early under the tongue.
- If available, oxygen can be given by face mask at a flow rate of 5–10 litres/minute.
- This treatment of a heart attack has been summarised as MONA (morphine, oxygen, nitrate spray, aspirin).
- If the heart attack leads to complete collapse then start basic life support with chest compressions (as above).
- Failure of the heart to restart from an irregular rhythm may require rapid defibrillation with an AED.

Occasionally severe acid indigestion with reflux can be confused with cardiac pain. To help distinguish the two,

**Chest disorders**

there is usually a history of reflux and the symptoms respond to antacids such as Gaviscon or a glass of milk.

> **Early evacuation.** A patient who has suffered a heart attack will need further management and requires early evacuation.

---

**AT A GLANCE – Heart attack**
- Administer drugs as per MONA
  Morphine
  Oxygen
  Nitroglycerin spray (or sublingual tablets)
  Aspirin

Epilepsy is caused by abnormal activity in the brain. An epileptic fit can be a scary experience to witness. There are many different types of epileptic fit but for the purposes of this handbook three will be described.

**Absence seizures**, previously called *petit mal*, occur typically in children and young people. They manifest as a period of vacancy and staring into space with a brief loss of awareness. Episodes of *petit mal* may last 10 seconds and can recur many times in a day.

Otherwise seizures may be **focal** or **general** and the patient will exhibit uncontrollable jerking movements of the arms and legs with loss of awareness or, in many cases, loss of consciousness. Focal seizures result in the involuntary jerking of the same part of the body, an arm or a leg, with every fit. A general seizure, or *grand mal* fit, can cause an abrupt loss of consciousness with body stiffening, twitching and shaking. A *grand mal* fit can lead to temporary loss of bladder control and to biting of the tongue.

### Treatment

The first line of treatment is to keep the patient safe and prevent injury to them or other members of the crew.

- Do not attempt to restrain them or put anything in their mouth. This manoeuvre was once advocated to prevent tongue biting but is no longer advised.
- The post-ictal phase is when the fitting has ceased but the patient has not regained full consciousness and usually lasts less than half an hour. As soon as the fitting has ceased, normally after a few minutes, place the patient in a bunk in the recovery position.

ACUTE MEDICAL ILLNESS

### *Medication*

People known to have epilepsy will usually take regular anti-epileptic medication. Care should be taken not to miss any doses and so increase the risk of seizures. Epileptics may carry their own emergency drugs. A common option is Buccolam (10mg of midazolam liquid administered buccally that is inside the cheek) which will help terminate a seizure. Another benzodiazepine used to terminate fitting is diazepam 20mg administered rectally or 10mg intramuscularly into the front or outer aspect of the thigh. Intravenous injection is more effective but difficult in a fitting patient.

**Early evacuation.** If this is a first fit or there are multiple repeated fits or the patient has been injured in a fit, then they require early evacuation.

# Stroke

A stroke can be manifest as a weakness in a limb or difficulty with speech and recognised using the acronym FAST. Pain is not usually a feature.

**Face** – does one side of the face fail to move properly and can the patient smile?

**Arms** – can the patient raise both arms above the head and hold them up?

**Speech** – is the patient's speech slurred and incomprehensible?

**Time** – to call for help

Symptoms affecting the face, arms and speech can indicate a stroke.

### Treatment

The immediate treatment is to place the patient in the recovery position with the paralysed side down and check the airway. If the patient is unconscious then turn them every 2 hours to prevent pressure sores (see Unconscious crew, page 24). If still at sea after 2 days begin to move the paralysed limbs passively. Even if the patient is apparently unconscious and unresponsive, talk to them as they may still be able to hear and understand.

In some cases early specialist treatment in a stroke centre within 4 hours can reverse the adverse effects of a stroke.

### Stroke

**Early evacuation.** A patient who has suffered a stroke that has reduced their level of consciousness or caused difficulty with breathing or with swallowing requires early evacuation.

# Abdominal disorders

Abdominal pain can be very difficult to assess even for a professional. Intermittent pain or colic suggests bowel contractions and may mean intestinal obstruction, which is more likely if there has been previous abdominal surgery. If the colicky pain is in the mid-abdomen it probably comes from the small intestine and if in the lower abdomen from the large intestine and colon. The latter can simply be a sign of severe constipation.

## Constipation

This is well known to afflict those on long sea passages. It is better prevented than treated. Sailors should drink plenty of water and eat fruit and vegetables. If these are unavailable consider adding roughage in the form of ispaghula husk (Fybogel), methylcellulose or similar. For the constipated sailor start with a stool softener, osmotic laxative (lactulose), then a gentle laxative (milk of magnesia) and then a stronger laxative that stimulates the colon such as bisacodyl or senna.

## Diarrhoea

This may be caused by the ingestion of contaminated water or food. Steps can be taken to minimise the chance but, even when careful, avoiding diarrhoea cannot be guaranteed. Avoid untreated tap water and drinks with ice cubes. Be careful of raw vegetables, lettuce and salads as well as under cooked meats such as chicken, burgers and fish.

When suffering diarrhoea take plenty of fluids as dehydration can creep up unnoticed and become a problem. Water with electrolyte replacement powders or tablets added in the prescribed dosage should be taken in cases of prolonged diarrhoea. In the recovery period avoid fats, caffeine, undiluted fruit juices and alcohol. Antimotility drugs such as loperamide may help symptoms. Antibiotics should be considered if the diarrhoea is bloody, associated with a fever, severe abdominal pain or distension or if it persists for two days or more. Ciprofloxacin is a good choice.

## *Acid reflux*

Known as heartburn, this is due to the reflux of acid into the oesophagus and pharynx (throat). Antacids are effective in curing or reducing symptoms. Chronic sufferers will carry their own favourite medication. If no antacids are available then milk is helpful or, as a last resort, a glass of very cold water may afford some relief. Sleeping in a semi-recumbent posture may help. Heartburn can mimic genuine heart pain but can be differentiated from it by the relief given by antacids.

## *Vomiting*

Vomiting at sea is usually due to seasickness (see page 6) but can occasionally herald abdominal problems. If the vomiting is 'projectile', a large amount that seems to fire out under pressure, it may well be associated with an intra-abdominal malady. Vomiting large volumes of foul fluid, like dishwater, together with abdominal distension suggests intestinal obstruction. Vomiting blood in any quantity indicates bleeding from the oesophagus, stomach or duodenum caused by inflammation or an ulcer.

### *Peritonitis*

Inflammation and infection in the abdomen is a surgical emergency. Initially local peritonitis occurs at the site of the affected organ (appendix, bowel, gall bladder, etc) but then becomes more widespread within the abdomen as generalised peritonitis. As well as abdominal pain, the patient is likely to have a fever and a tachycardia (fast pulse).

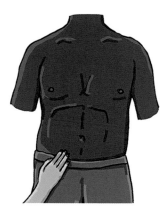

1  Lay the flat of the hand on the abdomen over the site of pain, for instance in the lower right quadrant over the appendix if appendicitis is suspected.
2  Press gently and if this causes severe pain under the hand, peritonitis is a possibility.
3  Now place the hand on the abdomen gently, as before, and ask the patient to give a small cough. In a case of peritonitis, this manoeuvre will also cause acute pain.

In some cases of advanced peritonitis the patient may be reluctant to cough at all and the abdominal muscles will

### Abdominal disorders

be rigid and board-like. If the signs are uncertain and the diagnosis remains in doubt repeat the examination after an hour.

The precise cause of the peritonitis, whether appendicitis, perforated duodenal ulcer, diverticulitis or other intra-abdominal disaster, is irrelevant as peritonitis cannot be treated aboard and the patient will need to be removed to a medical facility.

**Early evacuation.** Patients with persistent abdominal pain for 6 hours or more, especially if associated with projectile vomiting, a fever, abdominal distension and signs of peritonitis require early evacuation.

### Infections

Urinary infection in the bladder causes cystitis. Symptoms include pain on passing urine, frequency (increased rate of urination), urgency (a need to go immediately), cloudy foul-smelling urine and dull pain in the central lower abdomen.

To reduce the chances of developing cystitis, drink plenty of fluids and monitor your intake by watching the colour of urine. Respond quickly to the urge to pass urine, do not 'hang on'. This reduces the time that urine is stagnant in the bladder and thus more likely to become infected. Taking cranberry juice may help prevent cystitis. Cranberry juice may work by making the urine acidic and by inhibiting how bacteria adhere to the urinary tract cells.

Treatment of an established urinary infection requires antibiotics. A three-day course usually suffices. Co-amoxiclav or ciprofloxacin are suitable drugs along with copious amounts of oral fluids.

### Acute urinary retention

Acute urinary retention is the sudden inability to pass urine. It can occur in men of a certain age with prostatism, which includes many sailors. An enlarging prostate will lead to a poor urinary stream, frequency, urgency and nocturia (the need to go at night) and sometimes urinary retention. Certain drugs such as antihistamines and anticholinergics, which occur in drugs for seasickness, may contribute to making retention more likely. An unconscious patient may develop retention as can those with a severe urinary tract infection.

## Treatment

The treatment of acute urinary retention is to pass a urethral catheter into the bladder. Any boat that is going to sail long distance offshore with crew members who may be susceptible to retention must take aboard a catheter.

1 Before inserting the catheter, wash your hands and wear sterile gloves.
2 Squirt lubricating gel onto a sterile surface such as the sterile glove packet.
3 Wipe the urethral entrance and head of the penis with antiseptic. For a right-handed person, hold the penis vertically in the left hand with some traction.
4 Take the catheter with the right hand about 12cm from the tip, lubricate it with the sterile gel and insert it, gently advancing it up the urethra. The draining end of the catheter should be held over a container of at least 1 litre capacity.
5 If resistance is met, increase the traction with the left hand and ask the patient to give a small cough to help ease the catheter into the bladder.
6 When urine flows, the catheter is in place but must be advanced a further 5 to 10cm.
7 Now inflate the balloon with 10ml of sterile or bottled water and note that volume. Should pain occur on inflation the catheter may still be in the urethra rather than properly in the bladder – deflate the balloon and advance the catheter further before trying again.

The catheter can be removed after aspirating the 10ml of water from the balloon. Removal should be covered with antibiotic treatment continued for 48 hours.

# Gynaecological disorders

Pregnancy is no reason not to go sailing, but preferably stay near to land. It would be unwise to set sail at 35 or more weeks pregnant. If the mother is susceptible to seasickness, pregnancy may make it worse. The two main emergencies that would be of great concern on a boat are miscarriage and ectopic pregnancy.

## *Miscarriage*

Among those who know they are pregnant, miscarriage occurs in around 1 in 8. Women suffering a miscarriage are not always aware that they are pregnant although a pregnancy test will usually confirm it. When a woman begins to miscarry, the pregnancy test will remain positive for two weeks, even sometimes up to a month.

The main symptom of miscarriage is vaginal bleeding with red blood and clots. The bleeding may come and go over several days. Light vaginal bleeding can occur during the first trimester (first three months) of a normal pregnancy and must not be confused with a miscarriage. The common symptoms of pregnancy such as morning sickness and breast tenderness may disappear. The bleeding is often associated with cramping lower abdominal pain.

### Treatment

Miscarriage may require pain relief and fluids to replace loss. Some drugs such as ergometrine and oxytocin can reduce bleeding in a miscarriage but are unlikely to be available. Ideally the patient should be taken ashore in case of heavy blood loss.

Gynaecological disorders

### *Ectopic pregnancies*

An ectopic pregnancy occurs when a fertilised egg implants itself outside the womb usually in one of the fallopian tubes. Symptoms develop between the fourth and twelfth weeks of pregnancy. Lower abdominal pain on one side which can be persistent or intermittent is the main symptom. This pain may be associated with a brownish watery vaginal discharge rather than red blood. Changes in bladder and bowel patterns can occur but this may happen in a normal pregnancy too.

Rupture is a very serious complication of ectopic pregnancy. This will cause a sudden and severe pain in the abdomen along with dizziness or fainting from low blood pressure. Blood is lost into the abdomen and causes generalised tenderness especially in the lower part, symptoms that are indistinguishable from peritonitis. Vaginal bleeding may be minimal or absent.

### Treatment

Lie the woman down and raise her legs, treat with fluids and give pain relief to help relieve shock.

**Early evacuation.** A woman with a ruptured ectopic pregnancy requires early evacuation.

# Bites and stings

## *Insects*

Insect repellents such as diethyltoluamide (DEET) are extremely helpful. DEET should be applied in a concentration of at least 50% when it will last several hours. DEET 100% has been used and can last 12 hours but DEET 50% may be preferable. Much lower concentrations of 10% should be used for children under 12 years old. Do not apply insect repellent to broken skin.

**Highland midges** (*Culicoides impunctatus*) are found in the north of the British Isles, especially Scotland, in Scandinavia and Northern Europe. The midge is prevalent from late spring to late summer. The bite can be felt as a sharp prick often followed by an urticarial or raised skin swelling that is itchy and irritates. Midges prefer humid, damp conditions and are most active at dawn and dusk. Rain does not deter them nor does darkness. They do not thrive in hot, dry weather and tend to disappear if the wind speed approaches 10 mph.

To prevent attack by midges wear clothing so as to minimise the area of vulnerable exposed skin. Some sufferers go as far as to wear a midge net to cover the head. Midges will enter boats and tents so placing a midge or mosquito net across the companionway will help in the battle to keep them out.

Stings from **wasps**, **bees** and **hornets** cause pain, a stinging sensation, a red swelling and a rash. (Similar symptoms occur with stings from **jellyfish** and from certain fish such as the **weever fish** and **stingray**, both present in shallow waters.) A sting from any of these creatures can be intensely painful.

## Treatment

1 Do not touch the sting but remove it as soon as possible. This can be done by picking it out with tweezers. Otherwise cover the sting area with shaving cream or flour and scrape it off. This should remove the stings.

2 Apply a cold compress and sodium bicarbonate to ease symptoms. You can also soak the area in hot water, as hot as bearable – sea water will do. This causes the breakdown of venom.

3 Wash the area and apply a sterile dressing to any wound.

4 Local anaesthetic or ibuprofen gel will help the pain. Itching and irritation should respond to antihistamine (diphenhydramine 25mg, chlorpheniramine 4mg). If the inflammation is severe then consider hydrocortisone 1% cream.

### *Portuguese man o'war*

This is not strictly a jellyfish. It floats on the surface of the ocean and travels passively before the currents and wind. For this reason the creature can be washed up on the shore in numbers. It can still sting when grounded on a beach so do not handle one. It dangles venomous tentacles that are typically 10 metres long or more, even up to 30 metres. The sting is painful and leaves red welts and blisters on the skin where the tentacle has been in contact.

## Treatment

1 Remove embedded tentacle fragments with tweezers.

2 Rinse with vinegar and then apply heat using hot water, as hot as bearable, which should be effective in reducing symptoms.

**3** Hydrocortisone 1% cream will help soothe inflamed, irritated skin. If the skin reaction is severe and prolonged then consider oral prednisolone starting with a dose of 60mg, reducing daily by 10mg. Administration of painkillers (paracetamol with ibuprofen) and antihistamines (diphenhydramine or chlorpheniramine) may help.

## *Box jellyfish*

There are many species of these, some with tentacles up to three metres long, but the dangerous one, the Irukandji jellyfish from Australia, is tiny at only one cubic centimetre in size. A sting is extremely painful not just at the sting site but in the abdomen, back and limbs as well. The sting can be fatal.

### Treatment

The Australian Resuscitation Council recommends treating the sting with vinegar as this promotes the discharge of venom and prevents untriggered stingers from discharging. The patient will require morphine injection for the extreme pain, antihistamines for inflammation and even antihypertensives to control blood pressure.

Any of these stings can initiate anaphylaxis. The onset of symptoms such as skin redness, wheezy breathing, swelling of lips, eyes and throat, tachycardia and faintness calls for immediate treatment (see page 63).

## *Bites*

It is best to avoid bites, especially those from a shark, moray eel, barracuda, crocodile or dog. Apart from the obvious tissue damage, animal bites can lead to infection.

**ACUTE MEDICAL ILLNESS**

## Treatment

1 If unfortunate enough to get bitten, then wash the wound with soap and hot water.
2 Stop any bleeding with direct pressure (see page 29).
3 Soak the wound in hot water, as hot as bearable, for up to 90 minutes.
4 Do not attempt to suture a bite, leave it open.
5 Cover the wound with a sterile dressing and check daily for infection.
6 If infection occurs treat with a broad spectrum antibiotic (co-amoxiclav or ciprofloxacin). Everyone on board should be up to date with tetanus injections.

**Heat exhaustion** occurs with exertion in a hot climate. It is more common in the elderly, children, the less fit and those with a level of dehydration. Symptoms include dizziness, nausea, thirst, headache and muscle cramps. The temperature may a little raised but is often normal. The pulse will be rapid and the blood pressure low.

It is important to recognise heat exhaustion as it can progress to potentially fatal heat stroke. Treatment is to provide shade, splash with water, fan and rehydrate the sufferer.

**Heat stroke** can be fatal. The heat-losing mechanisms of the body fail and the temperature rises rapidly. As well as the symptoms of heat exhaustion, the patient may have a reduced level of consciousness or even be unconscious. The temperature may reach 40°C or more. The pulse and respiratory rate will be raised and blood pressure low. There may be shivering or fitting, the so-called febrile fit.

Treatment requires aggressive manoeuvres to reduce the temperature by fanning the patient while spraying and splashing with cold water. Total immersion in cold water will help. Apply ice to the neck, armpits and groins and, if available, administer oxygen at 6 litres/minute.

# Dehydration

Dehydration can readily occur on a boat, often initially unrecognised. When crew are cold, tired and sick, fluid intake is poor. Fluids can be lost through vomiting, sweating in hot climes and diarrhoea. To prevent dehydration, monitor the colour of urine. Should the urine become darker, do not ignore it, take a drink. An active sailor will require about two litres of water a day.

A combination of poor intake of fluid and excess loss will rapidly lead to a state of dehydration. Symptoms begin with weakness, lethargy, headache and eventually collapse.

### Treatment

The treatment is to take fluid and electrolytes in copious amounts. Proprietary electrolyte solutions are best. If these are not available make up your own. The formula is eight flat teaspoons of sugar to one teaspoon of salt in one litre of clean (boiled or bottled) water. Two to four litres may be needed in the early stages of treatment.

Consider the countries that may be visited and arrange appropriate prophylaxis and medication. This will mean leaving adequate time for inoculation as some vaccinations cannot be given together and may have to be staggered. For instance, if the MMR vaccine has just been given then a wait of four weeks is recommended before a yellow fever vaccination can be administered.

Certain vaccines such as MMR (mumps, measles, rubella), pneumococcus, meningococcus and others are nowadays given in childhood. For travel in the tropics, vaccinations are available for the bacterial diseases typhoid fever and typhus and similarly for viral diseases such as yellow fever, hepatitis A and B. Take expert advice on what is required for the places due to be visited.

## Malaria

Malaria is caused by the Plasmodium parasite and spread by the Anopheles mosquito. Malaria is a serious and sometimes fatal disease. There is not yet a vaccine. Prophylactic antimalarial drugs are not 100% guaranteed, so in affected areas, efforts must be made to avoid mosquito bites.

The anopheles attacks at night so maximum precautions must be taken between dusk and dawn. Wear long sleeves and long trousers. Place mosquito netting over the companion way, hatches and port holes. Consider anchoring in deeper salt water away from the shore. Use insect repellent DEET at 50% strength (less for children).

Antimalarial drugs should be taken before setting out and continued until safely away from the malarial area. The different antimalarial drugs vary in that some must be taken two weeks before reaching the malarial area and continued for a month after leaving while others can be taken for a shorter time. Some antimalarials are taken daily and some weekly.

In some areas of the world resistance to certain drugs has occurred, so specific drugs are recommended for particular areas. Drugs can have side effects, especially for pregnant women, so take expert advice before setting sail.

If malaria is contracted, symptoms may not appear for many weeks and often after the patient has come home. Any symptoms that occur on return from a malarial region, whatever those symptoms are, must be considered due to malaria until proved otherwise. Do tell the doctors of your voyage, do not leave them to guess.

# Poisoning

Poisons can be ingested, inhaled or injected through the skin, for instance by a bite or sting. For swallowed poisons, do not try to induce vomiting, which can cause more harm. For ingested fluids, such as acids, alkalis, detergent or bleach, administer copious fluids for example water or preferably milk. If ingested pills or drugs lead to loss of consciousness then start Basic Life Support (see page 19).

The greatest danger when it comes to inhaling a poison on board is carbon monoxide (CO) and to a lesser extent chlorine. **Carbon monoxide** can be given off by a poorly-maintained engine, generator or stove for heating or cooking, particularly if the exhaust or flue are leaking. The problem is worse in confined spaces with poor ventilation, like a boat.

Carbon monoxide is colourless and odourless so the patients, often asleep, are unaware of the gas and death can ensue. It is therefore unwise to sleep aboard a stationary vessel with an engine or heater running.

Patients suffering from CO poisoning exhibit lethargy, headache and loss of consciousness. The lips will be cherry red and the skin flushed.

When treating a patient of CO poisoning be sure to avoid the gas yourself. Move the patient to the deck for fresh air and check the airway. If available, administer oxygen at 6 litres per minute. If the patient is unconscious, place in the recovery position and if the patient has a fit, treat as for grand mal epilepsy (see above).

**Chlorine** can be given off when a battery bank floods and battery acid leaks. Sealed batteries are safer. Chlorine poisoning can also occur, particularly in children, from the ingestion of household cleaning materials.

Whether to evacuate a sick or injured sailor is not always an easy decision. Prior discussion with a medic to talk through the options can be very helpful. If within range of the coast, consider speaking to a local doctor onshore by telephone. Otherwise advice can be given by a medic via an MRCC such as Falmouth or else by a telemedicine doctor.

If near a harbour simply alter course to land the patient ashore and call an ambulance. It may be possible to call ahead for an ambulance either directly or through the Harbour Master so one is waiting on the quayside.

Transfer of a patient from boat to the quay, to a lifeboat, to a helicopter or to a ship is hazardous and must be done with care preferably by experts whether lifeboat men or coast guards.

If the vessel is further offshore and urgent evacuation is required then a lifeboat may be requested. The lifeboat crew will direct the transfer and many are trained as paramedics.

Should the vessel be further out to sea a helicopter can be sent. The range for helicopter rescue is about 120nm and when it arrives there is little hover time to transfer the patient, so be ready. Take instructions from the helicopter crew. Steer the boat on a straight course at a steady speed; for proper control, the engine is preferable to sails. Communicate with the helicopter crew via VHF.

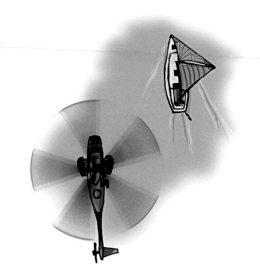

Rescue is usually from the port side of the boat into the starboard side of the helicopter with the wind on the port bow. The helicopter crew will drop a hi-line. Allow it to earth in the water or on the boat. Do not attach it to the boat or let it tangle with the rigging. Coil the hi-line into a bucket. A winchman will descend the line – be sure to follow his instructions.

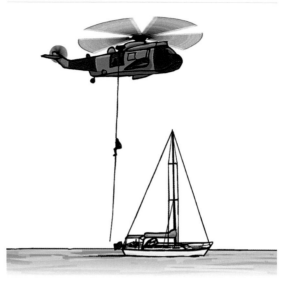

In rough weather it may be safer to recover the patient from the liferaft trailed astern. A patient that has been in the water for a period of time will be raised into the helicopter in a horizontal position. This is to prevent the flood of blood into the dependent legs that will lead to low blood pressure and even cardiac arrest.

When far out at sea it may be possible to transfer the patient to a merchant vessel or liner that may have been diverted by an MRCC. The ship may carry medical facilities. Such a transfer can be very hazardous and difficult to achieve. The sides of a ship are high compared to a yacht and the patient will not be able to climb a rope ladder or scrambling net. The risk of the yacht smashing against the ship and damaging her rig or her hull are high. If possible it is preferable for the ship to launch a boat.

# Reasons for early or urgent medical evacuation

The ease with which a patient can be evacuated will depend on the severity of the medical condition and the position of the vessel. Clearly evacuation from mid-ocean or high latitudes will present more difficulties.

### *Medical conditions for which evacuation is recommended*

Bleeding that is persistent and uncontrolled

Burns and smoke inhalation

CPR survivors (anaphylaxis, heart attack, hypothermia, drowning)

Epileptic fit if it is a first fit or fits are persistent and uncontrolled

Fracture of pelvis or thigh with blood loss or reduced circulation to the limb

Fracture of multiple ribs leading to respiratory distress

Fracture of the jaw

Heart attack

Penetrating eye injury

Peritonitis

Ruptured ectopic pregnancy

Severe asthma, especially in children

Stroke with compromised breathing or swallowing

Unconsciousness that is persistent following head injury or acute medical illness such as diabetes or stroke

## Medical kit

Assorted plasters

Bandages (crepe, triangle, sling, finger, adhesive)

Cling film

Clinical thermometer

AED defibrillator

Dental mirror

Dental filling (Cavit), dental first aid (Dentanurse)

Dressings (non-adhesive, sterile, hydrocolloid burns dressing, cling film)

Elastic strapping

Eye bath, dressing and eye patch

Finger bandage and applicator

Head torch

Intravenous fluids and giving set

Magnifying glass

Needles and syringes

Scalpel and blades

Scissors, forceps, safety pins

Space (foil) blanket

Splints (malleable, finger, hand, arm, inflatable, neck collar)

Sterile gloves (disposable)

Sterile wipes

Suture kit and sutures

Tape (micropore)

Urethral catheter (syringes, lubricant, drainage bag)

Wound closure (adhesive strips, skin glue)

## Drugs

| CONDITION | DRUG TYPE | DRUG AND TREATMENT SUGGESTIONS |
|---|---|---|
| Anaphylaxis | adrenaline, steroids, anti-histamine | Epipen (adrenaline), prednisolone, chlorpheniramine, oxygen |
| Allergy | anti-histamine | chlorpheniramine (Piriton), diphenhydramine (Benylin) |
| Asthma/ wheezing | inhalers, steroids | salbutamol inhaler, prednisolone |
| Diarrhoea | anti-diarrhoea, rehydration | loperamide, electrolyte drink, |
| Constipation | laxatives | ispagula husk, fybogel, lactulose, bisacodyl, senna |
| Dehydration | rehydration powder or tablets | rehydration powder or tablets |
| Eyes | antibiotic, eye wash | chloramphenicol eye ointment 1%, sterile saline |
| Indigestion | antacid | Rennie, Gaviscon, omeprazole |
| Infection (bacterial) | antibiotic | amoxicillin, flucloxacillin, co-amoxiclav, clarithromycin, doxycycline, metronidazole |

| Pain | analgesia | paracetamol, codeine, aspirin, tramadol, fentanyl, morphine |
| --- | --- | --- |
| | anti-inflammatory | ibuprofen, diclofenac |
| | local anaesthetic | lignocaine |
| Personal medication | diabetes, asthma, epilepsy, heart disease, lung disease, hypertension, allergies | various, prescription medications supplied by crew member |
| Seasickness | anti-emetic | cyclizine, meclizine, cinnarizine, hyoscine (tablet or patch), prochlorperazine |
| Skin | creams, lotion | calamine lotion, hydrocortisone 1% cream, co-trimoxazole 1% (canestan) cream |
| Sunburn | creams, clothing | hat and shirt, sunblock, calamine lotion |
| Bites and stings | anti-histamines and steroid cream, insect repellent | hydrocortisone 1% cream, anti-histamines as above, DEET (50% minimum) preparations |
| Wounds | antiseptic | sterile saline, chlorhexidine solution |
| Urinary retention | lubricant for urinary catheter | KY jelly |

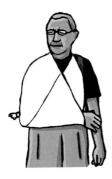

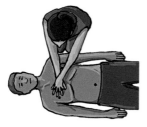

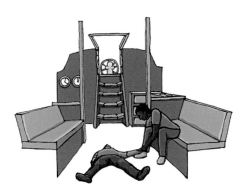

## OTHER BOOKS IN THE SERIES

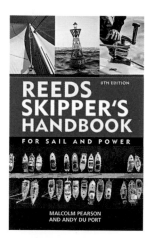

### REEDS SKIPPER'S HANDBOOK

Andy Du Port and Malcolm Pearson

*Completely revised 8th edition*

ISBN: 978-1-3994-1429-6

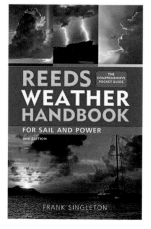

### REEDS WEATHER HANDBOOK

Frank Singleton

*2nd edition*

ISBN: 978-1-4729-6506-6